Dedications

'To my children Luke and Lauryn

for your growing inspiration'

Kids Backs 4 The Future (KB4TF), created for a
healthier lifestyle

© Written By Lyndee M Oscar

ISBN-13:978-1519268853

Illustrated by Shermain Philip

*"As a registered osteopath for over 23 years, it
is my responsibility to use my knowledge of
back care to protect the younger generation
from unnecessary musculoskeletal risk.
Prevention is always better than cure"*

Lyndee M.Oscar MSc., BSc (Hons)., D.O.

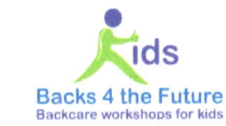

Backs 4 the Future
Backcare workshops for kids

www.kidsbacks4thefuture.co.uk

Founder of KB4TF
Helping Kids Become Back Wise!

Foreword

"Back pain is now the world's leading cause of human disability and together with related musculoskeletal conditions, accounts for a quarter of UK sickness absence. Orienting children towards positive health-related beliefs and behaviours is undoubtedly the most legitimate activity of our public health responsibility. Whatever good we can do for health is best achieved in childhood.
 This book gives children a good emphasis on physical activity as well as a physical awareness approach"

Dr Adam Al-Kashi, Head of Research and Education for BackCare – the UK's national back and neck pain charity

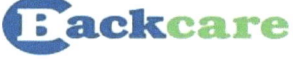

Our Penstripe back health page in school planners/reading books are supporting Backcare and Kids Backs 4 The Future in helping raise awareness of back care at school age

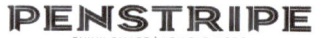

"In our modern world little, attention is paid to the damage caused to developing bones by modern lifestyles. Teaching schoolchildren to be aware of the impact ordinary activities in their daily lives can have on their bodies is vitally important to ensuring our children grow up with healthy backs. This book is a fantastic addition to any school library to inform children at an early age, before the developing bones in the spine and muscles are damaged from activities such as poor postures, reduced activity and carrying loads incorrectly"

Janet Fay Director

Marathon School Bag Specialist

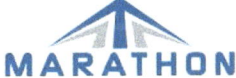

Sportsafe UK are pleased to support Kids Backs 4 The Future in keeping kids active.

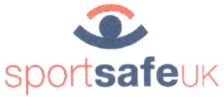

This is a play and learn book about our bones.

Every move we make, we use our bones and muscles *(say: Mus- els).* Muscles are all around our body and help us to move around. Muscles are attached to our bones by tendons *(say:Ten-dons)* and ligaments, *(say: Lig a-ments)* which attach our bones together.

Our bones keep us standing up straight, give us shape and protect our organs. Our brain sends messages to the muscles to move our bones. Our bones develop and change as we grow.

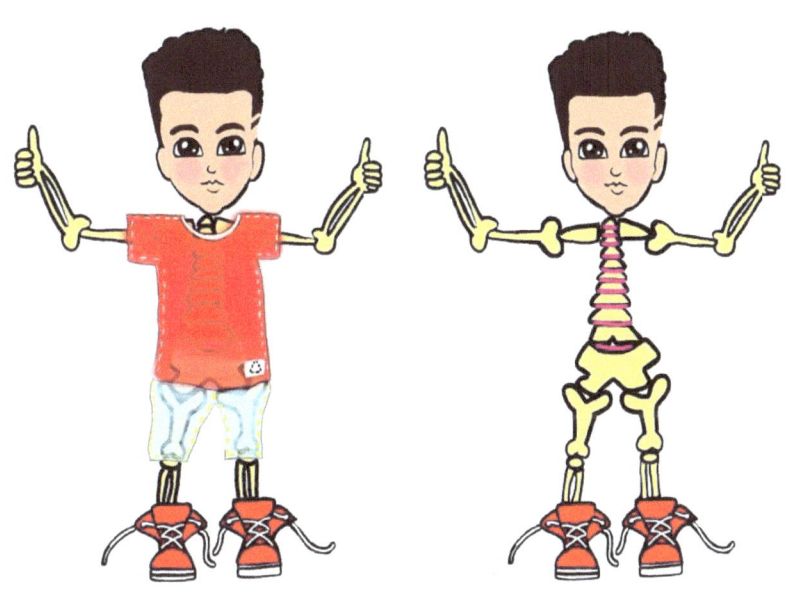

Our Skeleton

Our skeleton has 206 bones

Feel the shape of the bones in your hands.

Feel the shape of your ribs.

They are different shapes and sizes.

Imagine how floppy we would be without bones.

Our bones can keep growing until we are about 20.

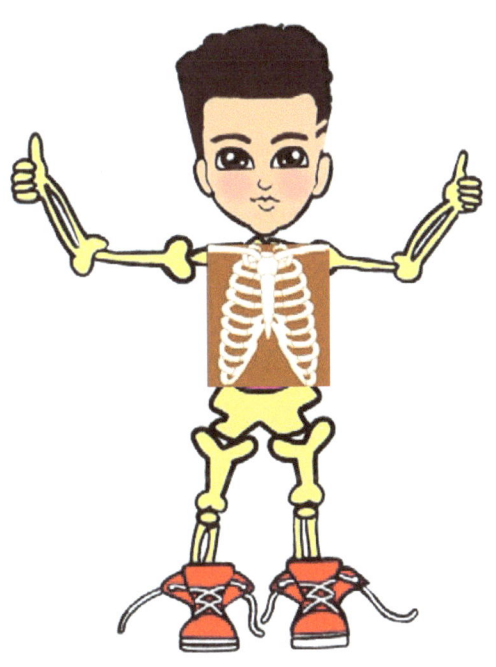

How our bones grow

Our bones need various vitamins, especially vitamin D, calcium and sunshine to grow.

Foods that have a lot of vitamin D and calcium in them are milk, eggs and cheese.

How do you get your vitamin D and calcium each day?

We must eat well to grow well.

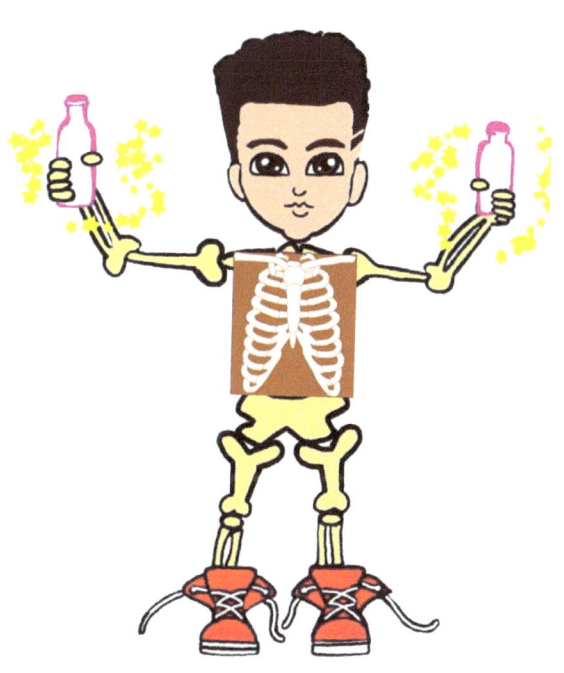

Our Spine

The bones in our spine are called the vertebrae

(say: ver tea-bray).

Our spine is also called our backbone.

The different curves of our spine keeps us upright in an

S shape curve.

There are **3** natural curves in our spine.

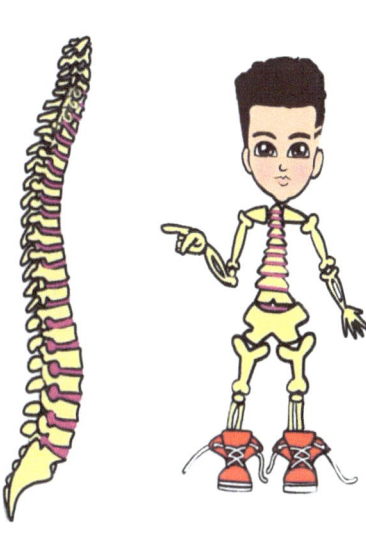

The top 7 vertebrae are called the cervical *(say: ser vi-kal).*

They support our head and neck (curve 1)

The next 12 vertebrae are called the thoracic *(say: thor ask-ik)*

They support our ribs and chest

(curve 2)

The next 5 vertebrae are called the lumbars

(say: lum-bar)

They support our low back (curve 3)

The different shapes allow different movements.

The big bone at the bottom is called the sacrum *(say: say crum)*

Point to your sacrum!

The final bone is the tip of the sacrum. It is called the coccyx *(say:kok- siks).* This bone is also known as the tail bone.

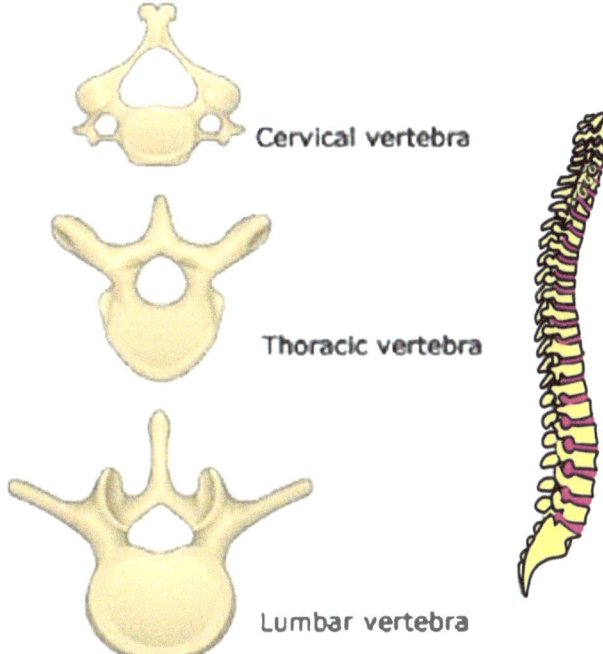

Cervical vertebra

Thoracic vertebra

Lumbar vertebra

Spinal cord and Nerves

There is a hole through each of the vertebrae where the spinal cord runs from the brain to the bottom of the spine.

The spinal cord and the brain make up the Central Nervous System.

The brain and spinal cord send out messages through the nerves telling the muscles and bones what to do.

These nerves branch out at every level of the spinal cord.

We all have cervical,thoracic and lumbar nerves.

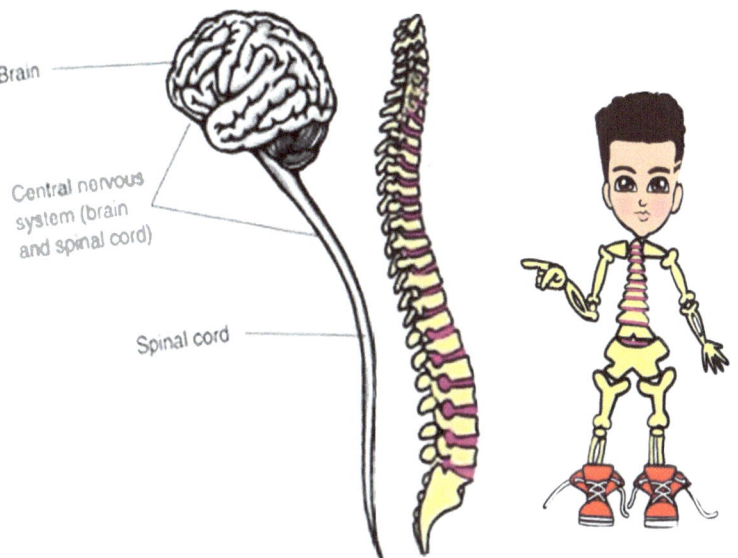

Brain

Central nervous system (brain and spinal cord)

Spinal cord

Strong discs

In between each vertebrae there is a disc, which is made of cartilage (say: kar-til-laj)

(Look at the pink areas)

The discs act like cushions so the bones don't rub together.

These discs are very strong and allow us to move about in many different ways.

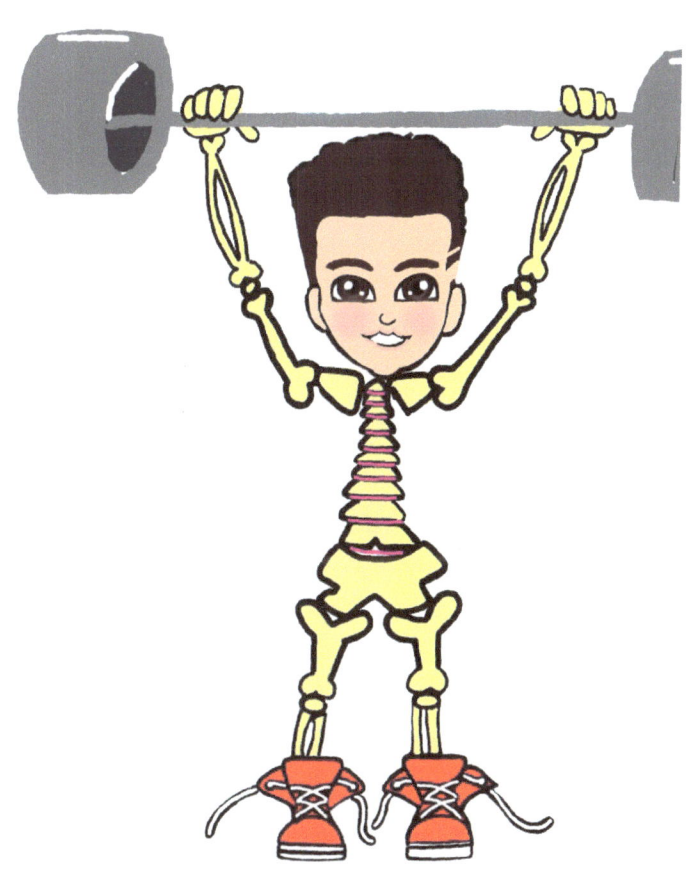

Cookies and marshmallows

Imagine putting a marshmallow in-between two cookies and squeezing it to one side. Look what happens, it bulges on one side.

When we sit crookedly and carry things on one side for a long time, the discs can also bulge and pinch on the spinal nerves, causing pain.

Ouch!

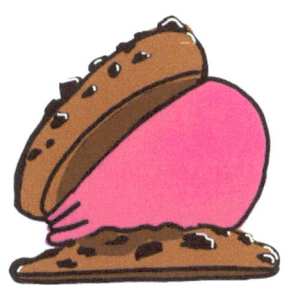

Look!

Look what happens to our spine when we carry our schoolbag on one shoulder.

We are making our spine crocked and bent to one side.

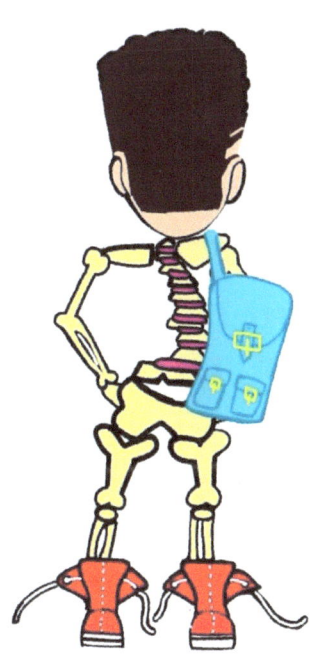

Look!

Look what happens to our spine when we are slouching when gaming or sitting.

We are making our spine crocked and bent to one side.

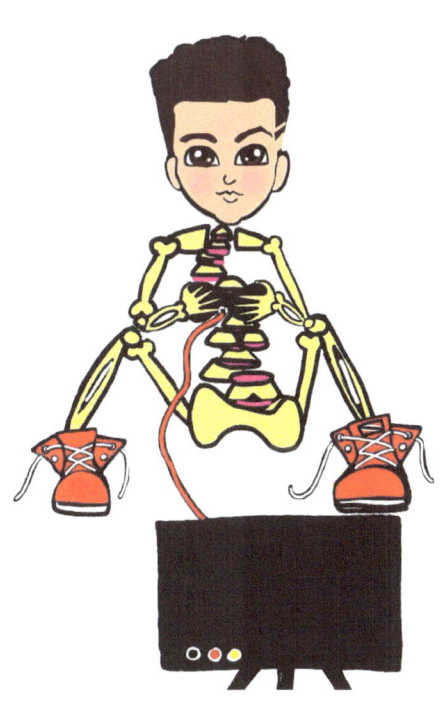

Ouch I'm in pain!

Doing these things often

**can make our neck and
back muscles weak.**

**Which can cause aches and
pains,**

and can make us feel tired.

**This can give us back ache,
neck aches and headaches.**

**It can also make our Spine
grow crookedly.**

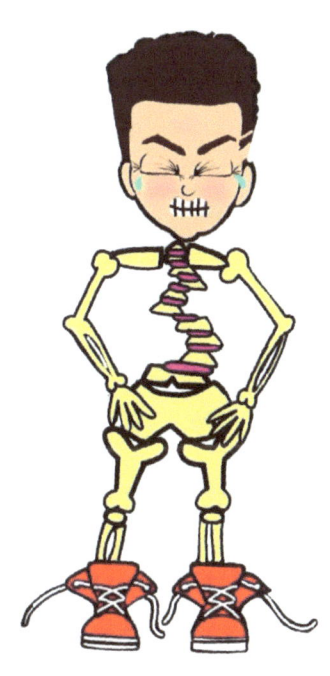

What we can do to keep our discs strong and our spine healthy!

Sitting up straight when we are gaming or on our laptop keeps our discs strong.

To help us sit upright, balance a single book on our head when sitting, watching TV or gaming.

Try it now!

Moving around, stretching out and not staying still in the same position for a long time will help our spine stay strong.

Use 2 straps when carrying our bag to keep our body balanced.

Eat healthy and get enough sleep to grow and stay well.

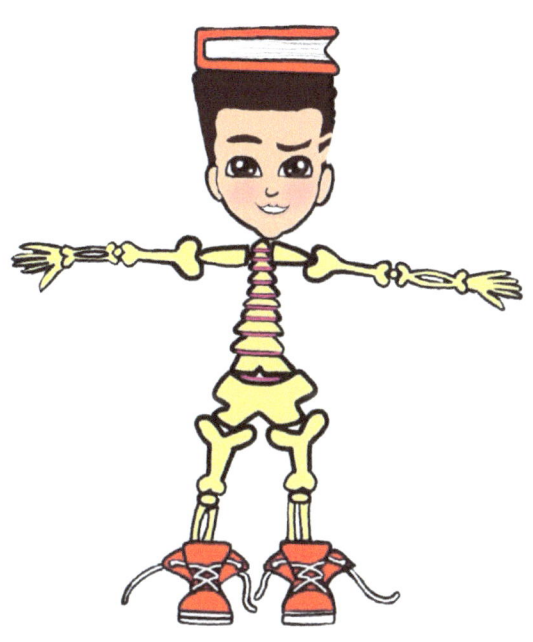

Remember

Keep active, stay positive, eat well to grow well and keep our body balanced.

Keep our spine strong by being Back Wise.

Exercises makes us feel good, relaxes our muscles and helps gets rid of stress.

Practice Today Prevent Back Pain Tomorrow!

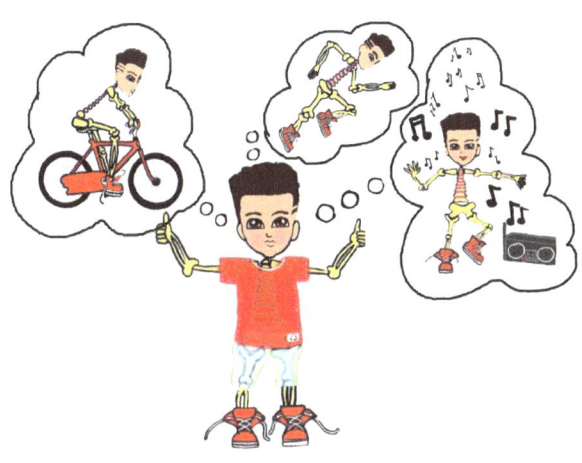

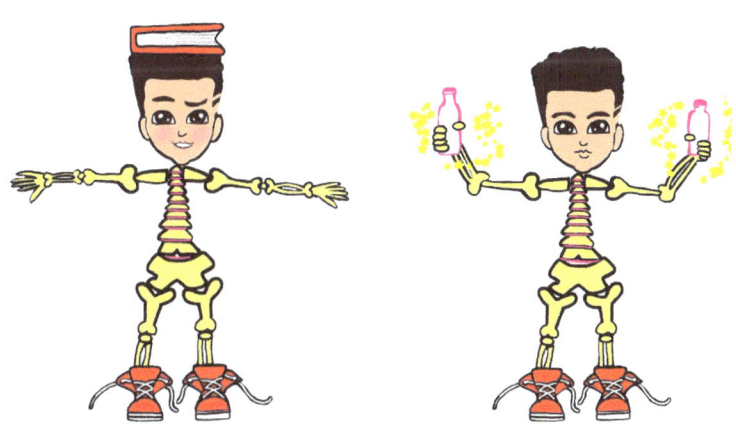

10 play and learn things to do after reading this book

Find the answers in the book

1. Our spine- What are the bones in our spine called? Point to any part of your spine.
2. How many natural curves in the spine? Can you point to them?
3. Our vertebrae- How many vertebrae in your neck? Count it out aloud.
4. Our discs – Where are your discs? What can you do to keep your discs strong?
5. Ligaments – What do ligaments attach together? Point to any ligament!
6. Tendons – What do tendons attach together? Point to any tendon!
7. Cartilage- What part of the spine is made of cartilage?
8. Nerves send messages all around your body telling your body what to do-What makes up the Central Nervous System?Point to these areas!
9. What does exercises do? What exercises do you do?
10. What can you do to keep your spine healthy? Show us!

Well done! Do these things to stay Back Wise!

For more support to help you stay Back Wise download our Back Wise posters www.kidsbacks4thefuture.co.uk

Also in the series!

Look out for

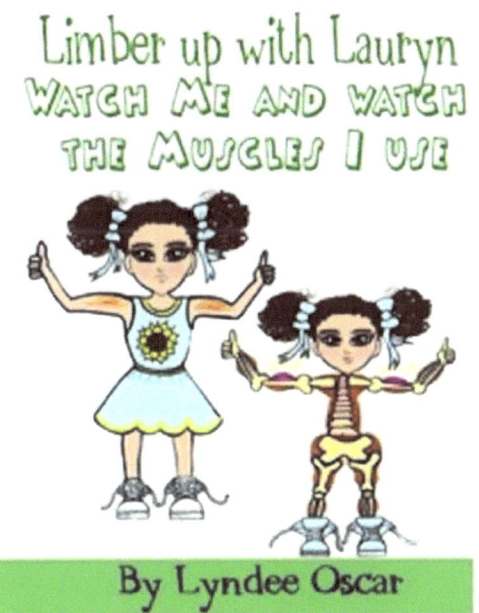

Limber up with Lauryn
WATCH ME AND WATCH
THE MUSCLES I USE

By Lyndee Oscar

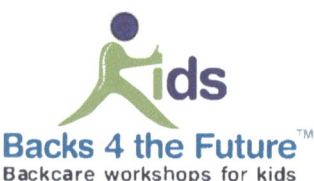

Kids achieve an A+ in being Back Wise

Backs 4 the Future™
Backcare workshops for kids

www.kidsbacks4thefuture.co.uk

SIT WELL

An **S shape** posture is a good healthy posture. It will improve what you do and reduce any pain or discomfort.

STRETCH WELL

Remember to take short regular breaks. Stand up, stretch out your back and hand muscles to avoid discomfort and stiffness. Adjust your position often.

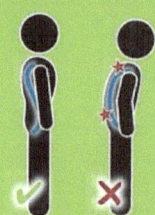

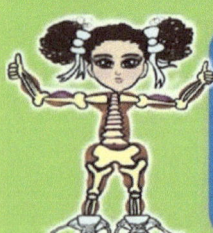

and remember to..
FEEL WELL!!
Keeping active, exercising and eating healthy will help you to grow well!

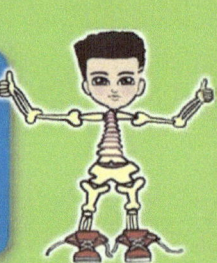

READ WELL

Keep your head upright and avoid looking down at your book, tablet or smart device as this will cause pain in your neck, shoulders and back.

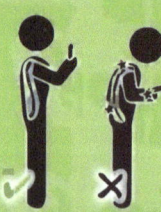

CARRY WELL

Keep your body balanced, stand or sit upright and carry your bag on both shoulders.

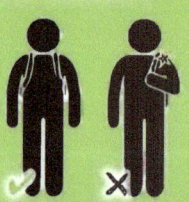

- **Practice these Back Wise tips today to prevent back pain tomorrow**
- **Keep Active**

- **Eat and drink well to grow well**
- **Keep happy**
- **Let someone know if you have back pain**

In support of 2015 **Backcare** National Awareness Class Campaign focussing on back pain in young people

CHAPTER 1: THE STRESS RESPONSE

In order to understand how the class of herbs known as adaptogens affect the body, it is import to understand what stress is. Most of us have used the term "being stressed" before. How often have you said, " I am stressed?" Most of us say this without knowing what stress is or what we really mean by it.

One of the first researchers in the field of stress was Dr. Hans Selye. He was the first to demonstrate, back in 1936, that stress "is not a vague concept, somehow related to the decline in the influence of traditional codes of behavior, dissatisfaction with the world, or rising cost of living, but rather that it is clearly a definable biological and medical phenomenon whose mechanisms can be objectively identified." [Selye 1985]

Even though people speak about stress in a vague way, it has a tangible form. Stress is a very real thing that is manifested in measurable changes in the body. The way the body reacts to the stress is very predictable with the key players being the hypothalamus, pituitary gland, and the adrenal glands. These glands are considered by many to be the principal effectors in transmitting and amplifying the stress signal [Seely and Singh, 2007].

5

The physiology of stress is very complex and beyond the scope of this book. However, some understanding is required to continue. Stress is managed by two different physiological systems: the hypothalamic-pituitary-adrenals (HPA) axis and the sympathoadrenal system (SAS). The SAS acts as the interface between sympathetic nervous system and the adrenal glands.

The stress response in the body begins with the stressor. This is sometimes referred to as the first mediator. This can be anything such as heat, cold, running up the stairs, emotions, and so on. This stressor immediately interacts with the limbic system in the brain, particularly the hippocampus and the amygdala which through the cerebral cortex sends messages to the HPA and the SAS.

The hypothalamus is often referred to as the "Master Switchboard." Once the stressor acts upon it, two basic things happen. First the hypothalamus releases corticotropin-releasing hormone (CRH). This travels through the blood stream to the pituitary gland. There, it stimulates the pituitary to further release adrenocorticotropic hormone (ACTH). ACTH triggers the adrenal cortex to release a series of hormones called glucocorticoids. The primary glucocorticoid is cortisol. At the same time, the hypothalamus, via the sympathetic nervous system, triggers the adrenal medulla to release catecholamine such as adrenaline or noradrenaline. This is the so called flight or fight response. Together the glucocorticoids and catecholamines cause physiological, biochemical, and behavioral changes in the body. These changes are known simply as the Stress Response.

There are many hormones that are released during the stress response, but the main one is cortisol. No matter if the source of the stress is physical or psychological, cortisol secretion increases with stress. Once secreted, cortisol begins to breakdown muscle proteins into amino acids. The liver converts the amino acids into glucose through a process called gluconeogenesis. This increase of glucose is used to provide energy for the brain. As cortisol levels increase in the body, more glucose is used by the brain. Simultaneously, the amount of glucose used by the muscles and other parts of the body decreases. The body switches to fatty acids as a fuel source. Cortisol is not all bad. It has other functions in the body such regulating blood pressure and cardiovascular function. Also, in the right amounts, it assists the immune system response to infection and inflammation. As always, too much of a good thing can be bad. With prolonged stress, the increased levels of cortisol actually suppress the immune system. The symptoms of prolonged increased cortisol levels include hypertension, anxiety, sex hormone imbalances, insulin resistance, obesity, osteoporosis, insomnia, and polycystic ovarian syndrome [Winston and Maimes, 2007].

Prolonged stress can be unhealthy, but that does not mean that we should, or can, avoid stress. In fact, the only time we can be without stress is when we are dead. Since the dawn of man people have been suffering and benefiting from stress. Stress can be beneficial. There are bad stresses (distress) and good stresses (eustress). Dr. Hans Selye is among the first to document how the body adapts under stress and is accredited with the discovery of the General Adaptation Syndrome.

The general adaptation syndrome is something that athletes should know well (see figure 1). It is the principle that explains how they get better with workouts. The general adaptation syndrome is broken down into three principle phases: alarm, resistance, and exhaustion. Each of these stages can be defined by their underlying biochemical mechanisms [Winston & Maimes, 2007].

The alarm stage is the first response stage and is characterized by the hormonal response previously discussed. It is the immediate response to the non specific stress experienced by the body. If the stress is not so severe as to cause death, the body will respond through the HPA axis by releasing a cascade of hormones, primarily cortisol, DHEA, adrenaline, and noradrenaline. These produce several effects on the body including constricting capillaries, raising blood pressure, increasing the heart rate, increasing blood sugar, and decreasing the function of the digestive system.

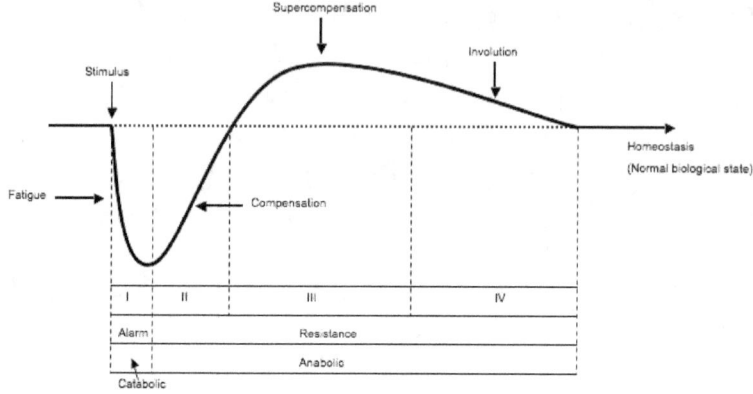

Figure 1: General Adaptation syndrome adapted from "Periodization: Theory and Methodology of Training." By Bompa, Tudor and Haff, G. 5th edition.

It is important to remember that this first alarm stage is an overreaction. The body actually produces more adrenaline than is needed to deal with the stress. If not used by physical activity, it can be harmful to the body. Too much adrenaline leads to surges in blood pressure that can ultimately damage blood vessels of the heart and brain increasing the risk of heart attack and stroke.

The alarm stage is considered to be catabolic in nature. During this stage, the body produces an excess of cortisol. Cortisol can break down the cells and destroy muscle. Many diseases and physical dysfunctions have been linked to prolonged elevated cortisol levels in the body. These include, but are not limited to, cardiovascular diseases, stroke, ulcers, and diabetes.

If the stressor remains, the body will move into the resistance stage. This is the anabolic stage, the stage of adaptation. The body adapts to resist stress and tries to deal with the stressors. For an athlete, this means with the appropriate rest, an increase in strength and performance will occur.

Healthy individuals usually can handle some amount of resistance unless energy is being wasted coping with an overload of stress. Prolonged exposure to the stress will keep the stress hormones at an elevated level. This will harm internal organs leaving the body susceptible to disease. Resistance continues to increase the cortisol levels in the body and decrease the production of DHEA.

If the body has enough adaptation energy, it will be able to adapt to the stress, and the body will return to homeostasis, or a normal stable condition. If not, it will continue into the exhaustion stage. By this time, the stress has been around for some time. The body has lost its ability to adapt to the stresses being applied. This stage has for some time been referred to as adrenal fatigue. Either way, exhaustion will lead to fatigue, immune system dysfunction, and ultimately death. For an athlete the exhaustion stage is often referred to as overtraining syndrome. This means the end of their season, or, in extreme cases, their career. If exhaustion continues, death will occur.

Wayne A. Pedranti

CHAPTER 2: ADAPTOGENS

Adaptogens are a group of natural substances that have the amazing ability to help the body adapt to stress, restore balance in the body, and support metabolic function. Adaptogens are unique in their ability to restore the balance of endocrine hormones, modulate the immune system and allow the body to maintain a heightened homeostasis[1] known as heterostasis. The knowledge of adaptogens dates back thousands of years to ancient China and India. However, serious scientific study did not begin until the late 1940s when Soviet scientists began experimenting on the benefits of these substances.

The idea that a natural substance could be used to improve mental and physical performance in healthy people was actually devised by the then Soviet Union during the Second World War. The Soviets were experimenting with the stimulating and tonic effects of *Schisandra chinensis* with their pilots and submarine crews. The roots of this investigation stem from the ethnopharmacological studies of Komorov and Arsenyev in the far east at the turn of the twentieth century. They found that Nanai hunters used the berries and nuts to

---

[1] Def. *homeostasis* – the maintenance of a stable internal physiological conditions.

reduce thirst, hunger, exhaustion, and improve night vision [Panossian & Wikman, 2010].

Between 1950 and 1960 toxicologist Nikolai Lazarev began carrying out the first documented pharmacological studies into the physiological effects of the natural substances found in plants. He found that some plants contained natural substances that could put organisms into a state of heightened resistance allowing them to increase their resistance to stress and more effectively adapt to physical and mental stresses. These substances became known as adaptogens.

Lazerev defined an adaptogen as an agent that allows the body to counter physical, chemical, or biological stressors by raising the nonspecific resistance to such a stress. This allows the body to better adapt to stressful situations. Later, Lazerev's protege Isreal I. Brekhman gave a more formal definition of an adaptogen. He defined it as follows:

1. An adaptogen is nontoxic to the recipient;
2. An adaptogen produces a nonspecific response in the body. There is an increase in the power of resistance against multiple stressors including physical, chemical and biological agents;
3. An adaptogen has a normalizing influence on physiology, irrespective of the direction of change from physiological norms caused by the stressor.

All adaptogens should be non toxic. That is they should not be harmful to the person using it. There is not much to say about this requirement. It is widely accepted and self explanatory. It is important to know that there are many substances that have an adaptogenic effect but have the potential to be toxic. *Eleutherococcus senticosus*, *Rhodiola rosea,* and *Schisandra chinensis* are well known adaptogens and have been reported to be safe in acute and sub-acute toxicity studies. Furthermore, these adaptogens have been shown to increase resistance to highly toxic chemicals such as chlorophos, phosphorus, cyclophosphane, strychnine, analine, sodium barbital, hexenal, benzene and many others [Panossian & Wikman, 2010]. Adaptogens produce a "nonspecific response" in the body. By this, it is meant that adaptogens help in resistance or adaptation through the building of "adaptive energy" to keep the body balanced when affected by multiple stressors or other harmful influences. By "nonspecific response," it is also meant that adaptogens stimulate, activate, or promote a response in a nonspecific way. This is why the one drug, one disease paradigm does not work with adaptogens. It is interesting that one of the most famous adaptogens is ginseng. All ginseng have the genus Panax. Panax is derived from Latin and means panacea or cure all.

Lastly, all adaptogens have a normalizing influence on physiology. A property that is unique to adaptogens is the ability to influence the body's bipolar homeostatic balancing ability. Adaptogens are capable of returning stressed physiological systems to normal regardless of the direction of deviation. Adaptogens are bidirectional. They affect the body by both stimulating and normalizing several body systems simultaneously, including the neuroendocrine and immune system. In short adaptogens can reduce the activity of a hyper-functioning system and stimulate a hypo-functioning system. A good example of this is *Panax ginseng* (Asian Ginseng). Among this herb's active constituents are chemicals called ginsenosides. In particular, it contains ginsenosides Rg1 and Rb1. The first can stimulate the nervous system while the latter calms it. This is the bidirectional property that is common in all adaptogens.

In contrast, many drugs and herbs work in a unidirectional manner. With use of these unidirectional substances there is a potential to worsen preexisting disorders in certain individuals. Adaptogens are rarely given for one therapeutic action only.

Wayne A. Pedranti

CHAPTER 3: THE STIMULATING EFFECT OF ADAPTOGENS.

Early studies on adaptogens by the Russians was primarily directed at increasing the mental and physical working capacity in workers. These early studies were directed at evaluating the response following a single or repeated dose in humans and animals. Substances of these types are usually referred to as stimulants. However, adaptogens differ considerably from this group.

The ability of stimulants such as caffeine, nicotine, and amphetamines to increase alertness and work capacity after a single dose has been well documented. However, they do it at a price. Stimulants tend to work by increasing the release of stress hormones, especially adrenaline and cortisol. This increase in hormone release increases the activity in the sympathetic nervous system, and is almost always followed by fatigue. This is often referred to as "the crash." This usually results in repeated doses of the stimulant of choice. Long term use of stimulants can impair mental function, causes insomnia, nervousness, anxiety and ultimately adrenal depletion.

Adaptogens differ greatly in function than stimulants. They work more as metabolic regulators. They are nearly all tonic in nature.

Tonics strengthen and invigorate various organs and body systems. Many tonic substances continue to increase energy even after repeated doses, and leave a residual effect after the dose decreases. In order for a substance to be considered a tonic, it must have a broad and profound health promoting action with no negative side effects, thus allowing for long term use with cumulative benefits. An example of this is Astragalus. As a tonic, Astragalus has tonic effects on the immune system, but it also supports the respiratory and cardiovascular systems. It is important to note that all adaptogens have tonic effects, but not all tonics are adaptogens.

As tonics, adaptogens improve cellular energy production while helping maintain energy reserves. They stimulate the central nervous system in a totally different fashion than stimulants. They work as metabolic regulators. Unlike the stimulants, adaptogens actually enhance the recovery process after exhaustive physical work or exercise. They also lack the negative side effects of the stimulants. (see Table 1). Adaptogens stimulate and support the neuroendocrine system.

"Repeated administration of adaptogens tend to give rise to an adaptogenic, or stress-protective, effect in a manner analogous to that produced by repeated physical exercise, leading to prolonged state of nonspecific response (SNSR) and increases endurance and stamina under extreme conditions [Panossian and Wagner, 2005]." Repeated dosage of adaptogenic herbs have been shown to have an anti-fatigue effect. This can lead to increased endurance or to more rapid recovery from strenuous events. This has shown to be valuable to athletes. Furthermore, unlike the stimulants, as discussed earlier, these adaptogens not only inhibit the stress response of an organism, but actually help create an adaptive change in the organism as a response to the repeated stress-agonistic effect of the adaptogen. It is important to note that the stimulating (acute/single dose) and the tonic (repeated administration) effects of adaptogens are byproducts of their stress protective activity.

		Stimulants	Adaptogens
1.	Recovery process after exhaustive physical load	Low	High
2.	Energy depletion	Yes	No
3.	Performance in stress	Decrease	Increase
4.	Survival in stress	Decrease	Increase
5.	Quality of arousal	Bad	Good
6.	Insomnia	Yes	No
7.	Side effects	Yes	No
8.	DNA/RNA and protein synthesis	Decrease	Increase

Table 1: The Difference Between Adaptogens and Other Stimulants adapted from "Effects of Adaptogens on the Central Nervous System and the Molecular Mechanisms Associated with Their Stress Protective Activity." By Panossian, Alexander and Wikman, Georg Pharmaceuticals (2010) 188-224

The stress-protective effect of adaptogens have been demonstrated in vivo, in vitro, on simple organisms, and in isolated cells. Adaptogens directly affect the regulation and homeostasis of the neuro-endocrine -immune complex.

"In addition there may be a connection with more evolutionary older congenial mechanisms of regulation in the cellular homeostasis and the adaptive/defense response to external stressors."[Panossian and Wikman, 2010]

Pannossian and Wikman suggest that this type of defense system is common to all cells and living organisms and probably includes heat shock proteins among other mediators.

Wayne A. Pedranti

CHAPTER 4: ADAPTOGENS AND THE ATHLETE

Although studies have shown that adaptogens are useful in the treatment of many stress related disorders, one of the most researched aspects of the use of adaptogens has been in the area of sports medicine and physiological performance.

Using the principles of the General Adaptation Syndrome, athletes often go far into the resistance phase, and sometimes into the exhaustion phase. With the proper rest, this repetitive loading can lead to super restoration. In other words we get stronger. However, if the proper rest, or removal of the stress, is not achieved, performance of the athlete can be reduced. This is known as over training syndrome.

As training volume and/or intensity increases, so does the physiological stresses on the body. These added stresses force the body to use its natural defense mechanisms to repair and replace any damage that has occurred. Adaptogens by their nature assist the body in making this defense system to work more efficiently. The result is that the body is able to adapt positively to the intense stress from exercise while delaying the exhaustion phase. This allows the athlete to train and race at a higher level.

The research done by the Russians showed that many adaptogens can increase the amount of ATP (Andenosine Triphosphate) and CP (creatine phosphate) in the muscle by increasing the levels of the fatty acids [Winston and Maimes, 2007]. ATP is the energy of life. It is used at the cellular level. The cells usually store enough ATP for a few seconds of work. It then uses the creatine phosphate for a few more seconds of work. After that it needs oxygen to make ATP. Increased storage of ATP means more energy for the athlete. Adaptogens also increase the amount of oxygen available for prolonged exertion by increasing the amount of oxygen circulated to the muscles and the brain.

The benefit of Adaptogens for the athlete does not end there. Other benefits include improvement in pulse rate and endurance. They reduce fatigue. They have a beneficial effect on the cardiovascular and respiratory systems. They have an anabolic effect because adaptogens aid in the rebuilding of muscle tissues resulting in increased muscle mass and strength.

The use of adaptogens by athletes is not a new idea. The documented use of adaptogens in the Olympics go back to 1972, and they are highly associated with the success of the USSR Olympic Team in 1980. By 1996 summer Olympics, 150 American athletes were using an adaptogenic formula based on the research of Dr. Brekhman known as Prime One. It is important to note that as of the release of the 2010 list of prohibited substances published by the World Anti-Doping Agency, no adaptogens were listed [WADA, 2010]. This makes it possible for athletes to use adaptogens with good conscience and without fear of testing positive for a controlled substance.

As mentioned earlier, adaptogens go against the one drug, one disease principle. Each particular adaptogen effect the body in broad, but slightly different fashions. We will discuss several popular adaptogens and the affects they have on the body. This will be followed by discussing how to combine individual adaptogens to increase the desired effects. The value of the use of adaptogens benefit everyone, but focus will be put on usage by athletes.

Wayne A. Pedranti

CHAPTER 5: ELEUTHERO ROOT (A.K.A. SIBERIAN GINSENG) – *ELEUTHEROCOCCUS SENTICOSUS*

Eleuthero Root is without doubt the most used and most studied adaptogen. This herb grows in northern Siberia and is often referred to as Siberian Ginseng even though it is not a true ginseng.

Eleuthero Root, as an adaptogen, is relatively mild. It may be used by men, women, children and the elderly. It is very effective over long term use. There was a study done in East Germany and Russia in the 1950's. There were 11,000 people in the study and 14 PhD's wrote papers on the subject. They all agreed by consensus that when 500mg of *Eleutherococcus senticosus* was consumed daily without let up that the subjects studied had 100% protection from every viral infection known to man [Ritchason, 1995].

Another study on the immunomodulatory effects of *Eleutherococcus senticosus* found that when an extract was injected intraperitonealy[2], cytostostatic activity of the natural killer cells increased by 200% after one week. A study on 838 children showed an increase in both T and B lymphocytes and 10 percent reduction in overall infections,

---

[2] Def. *intraperitonealy* – The act of administering directly into the peritoneum or the membrane that lines the abdominal body cavity.

including a 60 percent reduction in pneumonia [Monograph, 2006]. *In vitro* studies have shown that *Eleutherococcus senticosus* root extract inhibits the replication of RNA viruses.

The strengthening of the immune system is only one of the many virtues of this herb. Most studies have been in the field of athletic improvement. Modern research suggests that *Eleutherococcus senticosus* has the following effects on the body:

- It enhances muscle-glycogen resynthesis after exercise;
- It raises muscle creatine phosphate levels;
- It has a positive effect on "nitrogen balance";
- It has a stress lowering effect resulting in decreased cortisol production.

Muscle glycogen and phosphagens (creatine phosphate) provide a large amount of the energy required for high intensity training. As muscle glycogen levels deplete, there is a corresponding reduction in isometric strength and isokinetic force produced by the muscle. In other words the muscles become fatigued. If through the use of *Eleutherococcus senticosus* the resynthesis of glycogen is enhanced, then the athlete would recover quicker thus allowing them to perform several difficult workouts in a short period of time.

Phosphagens form the energy used in short duration high intensity exercise. ATP (Andenosine Triphosphate) works with CP (creatine phosphate) to provide the anaerobic energy for the first seconds of training. ATP gives energy for four to five seconds. After that, CP takes over. This lasts for another 5 to 6 seconds. After that, CP is used mainly to replenish ATP by giving up a phosphate. The free creatine over time is able to regroup into CP again. This requires oxygen and rest. It is clear that higher levels of CP in the cell directly influences performance. The higher the intensity of the workout, the higher the dependence on CP. Heightened CP levels increases the athletes ability to sustain high-intensity workouts over short periods of time.

About one fifth of our flesh consists of nitrogen. Protein of muscle is comprised of about 17% nitrogen. Creatine is about 32% nitrogen. Dr. Bernard Jensen, in his epic book The Chemistry of Man, described nitrogen as " the restraining element that balances the radical, explosive qualities of oxygen; it functions chiefly as a vitalizing agent and tissue constructor." If nitrogen metabolism is optimal, the individual is alert and intelligent. If nitrogen metabolism is less than optimal, the opposite is true.

Nitrogen is needed to synthesize creatine, niacin, and B12. Even DNA nucleotides contain one of four nitrogen bases: adenine, guanine, cytosine and thymine. Protein supplies the only known dietary source of nitrogen. Scientists use an index known as nitrogen balance to evaluate if there are adequate amounts of protein assimilated from the diet. It is a simple comparison between the nitrogen uptake and the nitrogen excretion. Prolonged stress, injury, illness, infections, and increased exercise volume or intensity cause the body to excrete more nitrogen than usual. This confirms that protein is used at a faster rate in these conditions.

If nitrogen excretion exceeds nitrogen intake, muscle is cannibalized for fuel to supply the needs of the body. This is what happens in many popular weight loss diets that result in muscle loss instead of fat loss. In order to regain lost muscle or gain new lean tissue, it is necessary to maintain a positive nitrogen balance. Maintaining a positive nitrogen balance allows the body to repair and rebuild muscle tissue, fight infection, recover from illness, handle stress, and stay well. That is why quality protein consumption is so important. By improving nitrogen balance, *Eleutherococcus senticosus* could possibly assist the athlete in building and repairing lean muscle and recover from strenuous exercise quicker than without.

Eleutherococcus senticosus, as part of its stress lowering abilities, reduces the release of the stress hormone cortisol. Cortisol has a catabolic effect on the muscles. It facilitates the conversion of protein in muscles and connective tissue into glucose and glycogen. By reducing the amount of cortisol being released after a stressful workout, *Eleutherococcus senticosus* allows the athlete to rebuild the muscle tissue more effectively after the training session due to the less protein being used for fuel.

An eight week study in China showed a significant increases in VO$_2$max, endurance time to exhaustion, and highest heart rate [Kuo Et al, 2010]. This same study also showed that the *Eleutherococcus senticosus* group had a significant increase in plasma free fatty acids and a decrease in glucose level. The study concluded that 800mg daily of *Eleutherococcus senticosus* enhanced endurance capacity, elevated cardiovascular function and altered the metabolism for using fat over carbohydrates as fuel in recreationaly trained athletes.

All of the active components of *Eleutherococcus senticosus* are at this time not clear. However special interest has been put on the seven Eleutherosides. The most important of these are most likely Eleutheroside B and Eleutheroside E. Eleutheroside B has been linked with improved protein synthesis, decreased stress and delayed fatigue in numerous studies. Eleutheroside E has also been linked to decreased Stress and fatigue

In summary, *Eleutherococcus senticosus* benefits athletes by increasing endurance and stamina, enhancing mitochondrial activity, speeding up recovery time, and preventing immune-depletion from excessive training. In addition, it has shown to be beneficial for nervous disorders and helps reduce mental and physical exhaustion. It improves mental focus due to the increase in cerebral circulation. It is a blood tonic and has been shown affective in treating early stages of atherosclerosis.

CHAPTER 6: RHODIOLA (ROSE ROOT)- *RHODIOLA ROSEA*

Rhodiola rosea is commonly referred to as rose root due to its faint rose like, fragrant odor. Rose root is native to the northern regions of Canada, Scandinavia and Siberia as well as the high altitudes of the Alps and the Pyrenees mountains.

Rhodiola rosea has been used historically by the Tibetans to nourish the lung and treat lung problems. In Siberia it was taken in the wet winters to prevent illness. The vikings used it to enhance mental and physical endurance. It was included in the first Swedish pharmacopoeia in 1755.

Rhodiola rosea, like many adaptogens, has many broad uses. Unlike *Panax ginseng, Rhodiola rosea* is a cooling adaptogen. This means that it is less likely to cause overstimulation. It has great benefits to the nervous system, enhances alertness, reduces fatigue, improves memory, improves depressed mental states, and protects the cardiovascular system. Like all adaptogens, it has a beneficial affect on the endocrine systems and helps balance blood sugar levels. Studies have shown that *Rhodiola rosea* can decrease symptoms of Parkinson's disease, relieve muscle stiffness and spasms, and enhance both male and female reproductive function when the problems are associated with stress or hormonal imbalances. Many studies on animals and humans has shown that there are many benefits for the cardiovascular system. It has especially been shown to strengthen the heart muscle. David Winston, Naturopath and author of the book Adaptogens, believes that it makes good sense for *Rhodiola rosea* to be part of any clinical protocol for people with Alzheimer's, cancer, fibromyalgia, chronic fatigue, immune deficiency syndrome, diabetes, and congestive heart failure [Winston and Maimes, 2007].

There are about 28 compounds that have been isolated from the roots of *Rhodiola rosea*. Twelve of these are compounds that are unique to this species. Most of the biologically active substances include organic acids, flavonoids, tannins, and phenolic glycosides. The two components most attributed to the adaptogenic properties of *Rhodiola rosea* are p-tyrosol and the phenolic glycoside[3] rhodiolaside [Kelly, 2001]. It is also suspected that additional phenolic glycosides such as rhodioniside, rhodiolin, rosin, rosavin, rosarin, and rosiridin may also play a critical role.

Of all the research on the affects of *Rhodiola rosea* on the human body, most were in the uses for treating asthenia. Asthenia is is a medical term denoting a feeling of weakness without actual loss of strength. It is characterized by symptoms such as fatigue, irritability, lack of appetite and sleep disorders. In 1975, a preparation of Rhodiola liquid extract was registered by the Ministry of Health of the U.S.S.R. for medicinal usage. This was tested on on 53 healthy individuals and 412 patients with neuroses, vascular dystonia, hypertension, asthenic type schizophrenia, and other asthenia[4] syndromes.

---

[3] Def. *phenolic glycoside* - A sugar bound with non carbohydrate functional group in which the sugars are in the simplest phenol form containing 6 carbon, and 5 hydrogen molecules.

[4] Def. *asthenia* – lack or loss of strength.

One of the surprising findings of this study was that the psycho-stimulating and adaptogenic properties of Rhodiola helped essentially healthy people that had some tendency to asthenisation when performing tasks requiring high mental exertion [Panossian and Wikman, 2005]. In these individuals, asthenisation showed itself in the form of reduced working capacity, difficulties in falling asleep, poor appetite, irritability, and headaches.

Further research done in the former U.S.S.R. confirmed the benefits of *Rhodiola rosea* as a treatment for conditions of asthenia. They indicated its use:

1. as a stimulant for healthy people in a state of fatigue and patients with asthenic states during the recovery period following somatic or infectious diseases;

2. for healthy people with a tendency to asthenisation during work requiring high mental exertion;

3. to recover working capacity during and after long periods of intensive physical work;

4. in cases of borderline nervous-mental disorders or neuroses.

Rhodiola rosea has been shown protect the body against stress induced damage and dysfunction in the cardiovascular tissue. It is known that when the body is exposed to extreme cold, the heart has a loss in cardiac contractile force. This phenomenon was prevented when an extract of Rhodiola was administered prior to the exposure to this environmental stress. In animals, after exposure to acute cold conditions myocardial contractile activity decreases. There is a partial recovery in activity 18 hours after the stress is removed. This recovery is considered partial because the heart tissue is not capable of stable contractability during perfusion[5]. A study performed on rats

---

[5] Def. *perfusion* – The act of forcing blood through an organ or tissue by means of the blood vessels.

found that in rats given Rhodiola prior to being exposed to acute cooling, the decrease in contractability was prevented and stable contractability of the heart tissue occurred during perfusion [Kelly, 2006]. Therefore, Rhodiola appears to have a beneficial adaptive response to this type of stress.

There is more and more evidence to suggest that during conditions of hypoxia and ischemic injury, that the vascular cells are impaired through the process of apoptosis, or the self-destruction of the cell. This can lead to an overall endothelial dysfunction. A study performed at the Chinese Academy of Medical Sciences found that when hypoxia was induced by cobalt chloride, that the level of apoptosis of the endothelial cells and intracellular reactive oxygen species generation was greatly attenuated when the subjects were pretreated with salidroside [Chu-Bing Et Al, 2009]. Salidroside is considered to be one of the main active constituents of Rhodiola. The conclusion of the study was that salidroside and *Rhodiola rosea* can protect against ischemic cardiovascular and cerebrovascular injuries.

Additional studies in Russia have found that Rhodiola was able to reduce stress induced heart damage. Stress induces the release of certain proteins and higher enzyme levels that can ultimately lead to damage to the heart tissue. Rhodiola prevented this release suggesting that Rhodiola has anti-stressor and cardio-protective benefits without harmful effects on the heart [Khanum Et Al, 2005].

Like many other adaptogens, *Rhodiola rosea* has been shown to have both anticancer and anti-tumor properties. Studies in this area have taken on two schools of thought. The first by the Russians is that Rhodiola can be used in conjunction with standard, conventional chemotherapy treatment. The second is that it can be used as a treatment on its own.

Rhodiola rosea is rich in phenolic compounds that are known to have strong antioxidant properties. Numerous studies performed on animals have shown that Rhodiola decreases the toxicity of common anti-cancer drugs such as cyclophosphamide, rubomycin, and adriamycin. At the same time, it enhances their anti-carcinogenic effect [Udinstev and Schakhov, 1991]. In their study, they injected two groups of mice with either Ehrlich ascites tumor or Lewis lung carcinoma. Both groups were treated with cyclophosphamide. This reduced tumor growth by 31% to 39% in both groups and limited the metastase of the Ehrlich Group to about 18%. However, it also reduced the number of leukocytes and myelokariocytes cells in the bone marrow by 40% to 50% and 20% to 25% of normal respectively.

On the other hand they found that if the mice were given an oral dose of *Rhodiola rosea* root extract following the transplant of the tumors, the tumor growth in both groups was suppressed by 19% to 27% and the Ehrlich metastases by 16%. The best news of all is there was no reduction in normal bone marrow cells. In the group that was treated with both cyclophosphamide and *Rhodiola rosea* root extract, the effect of the cancer drug was enhanced by 36%. There was also a reduction in the hepatoxic and hemeotoxic side effect of the cancer drugs.

Second only to the treatment of asthenic conditions, is the use of *Rhodiola rosea* for its general adaptive properties to non-specific stress conditions. In a study performed in the Netherlands on fresh water snail embryos, Rhodiola was found to have a strong protective action against lethal heat shock, the negative effects of chemically induced superoxide radicals, and heavy metal induced stress of copper and cadmium [Boon-Niermeijer Et al, 2000]. The heat shock group was exposed to 43 deg. Celsius for 4 minutes. The control group had a 9% survival rate, whereas, the group exposed to Rhodiola Extract prior to the heat shock had an 84% survival rate. The heavy metal and menadione groups showed a marginal increase in survivability as well. The group concluded that Rhodiola as an adaptogen enhanced the resistance to stress.

Like all adaptogens, Rhodiola has a positive effect on the endocrine system. In animal studies, *Rhodiola rosea* has shown to enhance thyroid function without causing hyperthyroidism. Rhodiola improves thyroid function by helping the body use energy well, stay warm, and keeping the brain, heart, muscles, and other organs working at their best. It also noted that the adrenal gland functioned with better reserve, and without the hypertrophy that is caused by normal stimulants. [Khanum Et Al, 2005].

In the 1970's, an experiment was made on mice in the Soviet Union. Sexually mature female mice were injected with rhodosine derived from rhodiola root [Khanum Et Al, 2005]. This was done over a four week period. They found that the menstruation was prolonged to 2.8 days as compared to the 1.5 days of the control group. This was accompanied by a decrease in resting days from 3.8 days to 2.2 days. They also found that there was a relative increase in estrus days from 29% to 56%. The experiments also showed that the rhodiola group had increases in the number follicles, the oocyte volume, the accumulation of RNA in the oocyte cytoplasm, the proliferation of the lining and glandular cells of the uterine horns, preparation of uterine mucosa for fertilization, and the weight of the ovaries. In other words, the mice became more fertile. However, it is important to note that there was little to no change in immature mice.

This led to clinical study on the role of *Rhodiola rosea* on women suffering with amenorrhea. 40 women with complete loss of menstruation were treated with a rhodiola extract. Normal menstruation was restored in 25 of the women, and eleven of them became pregnant. In a similar study showed that rhodiola substantially improved sexual function, normalized prostatic fluid, and increased 17-ketosteriods in the urine in men with erectile dysfunction and/or premature ejaculation. This confirms the benefits of *Rhodiola rosea* on the reproductive system.

Rhodiola has significant benefits for the athlete. It has been used for decades by professional athletes, including Russian Olympic champions, as a safe, effective, non-steroid supplement to accelerate muscular recovery [Abidoff and Ramazanov, 2003]. As we discussed earlier, *Rhodiola rosea* extract can increase both physical and mental performance by allowing the body to use muscular energy more efficiently. Russian athletes as early as the 1972 Olympics knew that Rhodiola would help them build up their muscular energy reserves. This enabled them to tap into their energy reserves when they needed it the most; under the extreme stress of peak physical performance that is required to win.

There are three main physical benefits of rhodiola supplementation for athletes that can be verified by over 100 studies:

1. It enhances muscle energy stamina during periods of peak physical stress;
2. It speeds cardiovascular and muscle energy recovery time;
3. It possesses pharmacologically relevant anabolic activity.

The effects of Rhodiola on the muscular energy system was made clear in a study on mice that were given 50 mg/kg *Rhodiola rose* root extract orally. The group treated with Rhodiola had a 24.6% increase in duration of exhaustive swimming in comparison to the control group [Abitov Et al, 2003]. What they found is that *Rhodiola rosea* extract activated the synthesis and re-synthesis of adenosine triphosphate (ATP) in the mitochondria. Furthermore, it stimulated the reparative energy processes after intense exercise.

In a similar fashion, a test was done on 14 trained endurance athletes. These athletes were given Rhodiola for 4 weeks and then given a cardiopulmonary exhaustion test. Blood samples were taken and compared to the same athletes after taking a placebo. What they found was that there was little to no change in the max heart rate, Borg scale level of perceived exertion, VO2 Max, or even the time to exhaustion. However what they did find was that *Rhodiola rosea* intake significantly reduced plasma free fatty acids, blood lactate and plasma creatine kinase levels. They concluded that supplementation with *Rhodiola rosea* will reduce skeletal muscle damage after an exhaustive training session [Parisi Et al, 2010]. A similar study done in Belgium on young healthy volunteers concluded that acute supplementation with Rhodiola would improve endurance capacity [De Bock Et al, 2004]. This means that Rhodiola has a positive effect for athletes in both short term and long term use.

Research on the effects of Rhodiola has been performed on many athletes including swimmers, skiers, speed skating wrestling, weightlifting, both speed and strength track and field, triathlon, gymnast, and the list goes on. All these studies (more than 180 since 1961) have either partially or completely supported the animal research. The general consensus is the *Rhodiola rosea* supplementation test subjects showed more robust pulse and arterial pressure, better coordination and improved recovery ability. Like most adaptogens, it is believed that *Rhodiola rosea* normalizes the autonomic nervous system and the sympathetic nervous system, which in turn optimizes performance and endurance.

One interesting aspects of *Rhodiola rosea* is that it appears to be void of unwanted side effects. When compared to other stimulants and anabolic steroids, Rhodiola does not have any negative effects on the adrenal cortex and endocrine glands. In a sense, Rhodiola is able to give similar benefits without the detrimental side effects on the adrenal glands. The L50 for Rhodiola is approximately 235 grams in a 70 Kg human, which is more than 450 times greater than the typical recommended dose.

The bottom line is that Rhodiola is a safe, effective herbal supplement that is able to give the user a competitive edge by enhancing physical and mental stamina and decreasing recovery time. Beyond athletic performance, Rhodiola has been shown to be helpful in cases of amenorrhea, depression, insomnia, asthenia, fatigue, topical periodontal disease, cancer, headaches, schizophrenia, colds and flu, hypertension, and impotency in males.

Wayne A. Pedranti

CHAPTER 7: SCHISANDRA (OR SCHIZANDRA) - *SCHISANDRA CHINENSIS*

In the East, *Schisandra chinensis* has been used for centuries, however in the West, it has only been used in the last 40 years or so. The Chinese call Schisandra wu wei zi. Roughly translated this means five flavors. The berry of the Schisandra plant is said to have all the five flavors traditionally used in Chinese medicine: sweet, sour, pungent or spicy, bitter, and salty. Staying with the Chinese tradition, these tastes directly reflect the five yin organs: the liver, the kidneys, the heart, the spleen-pancreas, and the lungs. In modern times, Schisandra is commonly used for ailments of these organs as well as its effect on the central nervous system and athletic performance.

Like all other adaptogens, Schisandra has very real effects on the nervous, immune and endocrine systems. As an adaptogen, Schisandra has a bidirectional effect on the nervous system. It functions as a mild stimulant enhancing reflexes, mental activity, and work performance. Simultaneously, it works to calm and relieve anxiety, as well as helping with stress induced asthma or palpitations.

The whole Schisandra fruit is considered to be salty by Traditional Chinese Medicine. Schisandra has a nonspecific effect on the endocrine system and an endocrine-mediated enhancement of the immune system. This is the part of the immune system most associated with stress. This part of the immune system is inhibited by chronic anxiety, anger, depression, and/or fear. People who suffer from chronic stress are more likely to catch colds, the flu, or other immune deficiency conditions such as cancer and chronic immune deficiency syndrome [Winston & Maimes, 2007]. In traditional Chinese medicine, the kidney-endocrine organs assist the lungs to fully inhale. The taste most associated with the kidney and endocrine organs is the salty taste.

According to Chinese medicine, the peel and flesh of the *Schisandra chinensis* berry has a sweet and sour flavor. This has, in their tradition, been associated with the liver and spleen. Interestingly enough, recent research has shown that Schisandra is hepatoprotective or antihepatoxic. In other words, it supports and protects the liver.

Studies have shown that Schisandra enhances the production and synthesis of a very powerful antioxidant in the liver known as glutathione. This antioxidant is sometimes referred to as the "Mother of all antioxidants" due to its beneficial effects on the immune system. It activates the detoxification of the liver. Schisandra seed extract has been shown to improve phase 1 oxidative metabolism in liver tissue damaged by CCL_4 (Carbon Tetrachloride). This is believed to be due to the presence of lignans with a dibenzocyclooctadiene skeleton such as schisandrin, gomisin A, deoxyschisandrin (schisandrin A), g-schisandrin and *wuweizisu* C. These components are believed to be active in the hepatoprotective, anti-inflammatory, anticancer, anti-HIV and immunomodulating effects of *Schisandra chinensis* [Wang, Rubin Et al, 2007]. Animal studies suggest Schisandra may protect the liver from toxic damage, improve liver function, and stimulate liver cell regrowth. These findings led to its use in human trials for treating hepatitis.

The modern lifestyle is associated with an increase in the incidence of fatty liver. Fatty liver is a condition in the liver characterized by a build up of fat in the liver cells. It is currently estimated that 15 to 20% of the general population have this condition, and the incidence is much higher in obese individuals. Fat in the liver may interfere with normal liver function and result in hepatocyte injury, hepatocirrhosis, or hepatocellular carcinoma. Fatty liver can also be associated with diabetes, tuberculosis, malnutrition, excess vitamin A, and even pregnancy. However, severe fatty liver is most often due to improper diet, alcoholism, and obesity.

A recent study in China found that an ethanol extract from the fruit of the Schisandra berry significantly reduced the hepatic triglyceride levels in mice that were fed a high fat/cholesterol diet [Pan Et al, 2009]. They found that the Schisandra extract could prevent or ameliorate the degree of liver steatosis in hypercholesterolemic mice without the liver hypertrophy associated with Fenofibrate. They concluded that Schisandra may be used clinically for the management of fatty liver disease and as a therapeutic option for patients with dyslipidemias, particularly those associated with diabetes, coronary heart disease, atherosclerosis, or metabolic syndrome.

The bitter taste of the Schisandra berry is associated with the seed. In traditional Chinese medicine, the bitter taste is associated with the heart. Schisandra has been shown to have an amphoteric or normalizing effect on blood pressure. It tends to lower high blood pressure and raise low blood pressure. It increases the contractions of the heart muscle and reduce palpitations especially when associated with stress.

Another taste associated with the seed is the pungent or spicy taste. This taste represents the lungs in traditional Chinese medicine. This taste supplements the function of the liver while nourishing the lungs. The pungent flavor has a "dispersing and moving effect" [Tierra, 1988]. Schisandra dries up excess fluid. It also has anti-inflammatory and anti-asthmatic properties that are beneficial to people who have asthma with wheezing wet coughs and chronic obstructive pulmonary disorder [Winston & Maimes, 2007].

Schisandra has many benefits for the athlete associated with its adaptogenic effects. It is well known that acute physical exercise (stress) activates the formation of cortisol and nitric oxide in the blood and saliva in individuals that are either new to exercise or sedentary. Acute physical loading does not increase the nitric oxide or cortisol production in the well trained athletes. In other words, as an athlete becomes more trained, the required physical loading increases. This is a direct result of the General Adaptation Syndrome discussed earlier.

Schisandra has a pro-stressor effect. In other words, it activates the formation of both nitric oxide and cortisol even in the well trained athlete. This activation leads to adaption to further heavy physical loading [Panossian, Wikman, & Wagner, 1999]. In a double blind placebo controlled study, athletes were given either Schisandra or a placebo. The athletes that took Schisandra before exercise had increased levels of nitric oxide and cortisol similar to the level of those that have undergone intense training. This correlates with increased performance. After training, the group that took Schisandra returned to normal levels of nitric oxide and cortisol much more quickly than those with the placebo. This shows the protective nature of Schisandra [Panossian Et al, 1999].

In another study, it was found that supplementation of Schisandra extract increased the swimming time to fatigue in mice [Cao Et al, 2009]. Schisandra increased the concentration of hemoglobin while preventing the increase in lactate and Blood Urea Nitrogen levels. This corresponds to a decrease in athletic fatigue due to over exercise and increases the time to failure due to fatigue.

In summary, *Schisandra chinensis* is a miracle adaptogen that works in synergy with *Eleutherococcus senticosus* for anti-stress, weight loss, and sports endurance. It has many positive effects in the body. According to Jack Ritchason N.D.[Ritchason, 1995] Schisandra:

- supports sugar levels and liver function;
- improves digestion of fatty foods by cleansing the liver and increasing the production of bile which then functions as a digestant for splitting the fat in the food to fatty acids and glycerin;
- allows the body to respond to stress more quickly, increase the body's capacity to work, and decrease fatigue. It increases blood circulation and bile production while decreasing blood pressure;
- increases the contraction of the heart muscle and uterus;
- increases the energy supply of cells in the brain, muscles, liver, kidney, glands, and nerves in the entire body;
- promotes long life of the cell;
- is capable of building the immune system and supporting the body against damage due to stress;
- has the capability to increase energy, strengthen the veins, and relaxing the muscles of the eye resulting in improved vision;
- protect against free radical damage;
- is helpful with coughing, lung weakness, asthma, night sweats, and prolonged diarrhea;
- balances body functions, normalizes body systems, and is effective in post surgery well being and recovery.

Wayne A. Pedranti

CHAPTER 8: ASIAN (KOREAN) GINSENG - *PANAX GINSENG* & AMERICAN GINSENG – *PANAX QUINQUEFOLIUM*

By far one of the most documented adaptogens is Ginseng. There are several varieties of ginseng, but the most popular are *Panax ginseng* (commonly known as Asian or Korean Ginseng) and *Panax quinquefolius* (American Ginseng). *Panax ginseng* has been used for thousands of years in China and Korea where it is used as a superior healing tonic. Some claim that Ginseng is the most effective adaptogen of all the tonic herbs.

Ginseng gets its name from the original Chinese name ren shen which means "man root" because the root is shaped like a man. The botanical name Panax is derived from the Greek work "panacea" meaning all healing. This name fits the herb Ginseng because it has historically been used to cure nearly everything.

Panax ginseng contains triterpenoid saponin glycosides[6]. These, however, are most commonly called ginsenosides. Many of the active

---

[6] Def. *saponins glycoside* – a fatty compound of hydrogen and oxygen that froths in solution like a soap. It is usually linked to sugars and contains essential oils.

compounds are found in all parts of the plants. These include amino acids, alkaloids, phenols, proteins, polypeptides, vitamin B1 and B2. However, the most active constituents are the ginsenosides. Through the use of thin layer chromatography and methanol extraction experiments, nearly 40 ginsenosides have been identified, twelve (12) of which have been identified to be the most active constituents.

Basically there are two different subtypes of ginsenosides: protopanaxadiol and protopanaxatriol. These are further classified by the arrangement of sugar residues[7]. Rb1, Rb2, Rc, and Rd are examples of protopanaxadiol ginsenosides. Re, Rf, Rg1, and Rg2 are examples of protopanaxatriol [Monograph,2009].

It is important to note that the concentration of ginsenosides is largely dependent on the age of the root and if the extraction is the red or white form. The red form is steamed after harvest and the white form is not.

Although Chinese physicians have been using Ginseng medicinally for well over 4,000 years, it is only in recent years that the research in to its use as a "Sports Tonic" has been done. Most of the research done with Ginseng has been directed to sick people, not athletes.

The best studies in the effects of Ginseng and ginsenosides on athletic performance have been done using a standardized ginseng extract to control the amount of ginsenosides in the formula. One of the most used is a standardized extract from Switzerland is known simply as G115 Extract. It has been used in numerous independent studies since 1971 [Colgan, 1993].

The benefits of Ginseng for athletes can be experienced in many ways. Ginseng can improve endurance, lift lung power, improve performance and recovery, and decrease reaction time. However, the

---

[7] The nomenclature of ginsenoside is by designation R_x, where X represents the retention factor value from the sequence of spots on the thin layer chromatography scale.

effects of Ginseng and ginsenosides extend well beyond these ergogenic, or performance enhancing affects. There is plenty of evidence that Ginseng helps regulate blood sugar, normalize blood pressure, improve glucose tolerance, aids the liver, and even causes apoptosis in cancer cells.

Ginseng reduces reaction time. In a double blind study performed by the Polish Academy of Sciences, 15 soccer players were divided into two groups. One group was given 350mg of Ginseng extract and the other a placebo. After 6 weeks of treatment both groups rode an ergometer cycle to exhaustion. The researchers concluded that the Ginseng group had a significant increase in reaction time (both at rest and during exercise) and an improvement in psycho-motor performance [Holly, 2007].

Ginseng improves endurance. One way Ginseng boosts endurance is by stimulating the brain and the adrenal/pituitary system to increase the production of excitatory hormones [Colgan, 1993]. These hormones increase the subjects alertness. In addition, other research has shown that standardized ginseng extract actually spares glycogen and increases the oxidation of free fatty acids. This means that the body can spare its limited sources of glycogen and increase the use of stored body fat. This should among other things increase endurance and improve athletic performance by delaying fatigue.

In one study, mice were put into a vat of water and forced to swim until they were too exhausted to swim any more and sank. After being recovered, the mice were treated with ginseng supplements for a few weeks. They were then put once more into the vat of water and forced to swim until exhaustion. The results were huge. The time to exhaustion increased by 40%, which is a large gain over what was already an all out performance.

Some lung functions such as vital capacity, forced expiratory volume, peak expiratory flow, and maximum breathing capacity are reasonably good predictors of athletic performance. In one double blind study, athletes were given 200mg of standardized ginseng extract or a placebo for 12 weeks. At the end of the trial, the ginseng group showed 44% greater improvement as compared to the placebo group.

This was confirmed by measuring the serum lactic acid at different work loads in athletes. Level of serum lactic acid relate to our capacity to use oxygen. As lactic acids levels increase, so does the amount of fatigue. Ginseng supplementation has been shown to significantly reduce lactic acid levels, thus delaying the onset of fatigue.

Ginseng has an antioxidant effect at the mitochondrial level. This is a good thing because 90% of all free radicals are in the mitochondria of the cells, and not all antioxidants can penetrate the mitochondria. These free radicals play an important role as mediators of skeletal muscle damage and inflammation after strenuous exercise.

The medicinal efficacy of *Panax ginseng* is closely linked to its ability to protect against free radical attack. Researchers found that the medicinal efficacy of *Panax ginseng* is directly related to its:

1. ability to prevent myocardial ischemia-reperfusion damage induced by hyperbaric oxygen;
2. protective effects against hepatic oxidative stress induced by exhaustive exercise;
3. protection against muscle injury and inflammation after eccentric exercise;
4. ability to inhibit lipid peroxidation through metal chelation;
5. ability to reduce the oxidative DNA damage caused by Fenton reagent;
6. and its ability to scavenge superoxide radicals.

Strenuous exercise increases the production of free radicals. Unfortunately, it is very difficult to measure the amount of free radicals directly. Therefore, it is common to measure them indirectly by measuring malondialdehyde (MDA) levels. Using this method, researches measured the lipid peroxidation levels in male rats after strenuous exercise [Voces, J Et al, 2004]. They found that all rats had increased MDA levels following exercise. The same rats were then treated with an extract of *Panax ginseng*. It was found that muscles after exercise showed a 74% reduction in MDA levels. This was irregardless of muscle fiber type.

Another aspect of ginseng that may be beneficial for athletes (particularly women) is its ability to naturally increase the production of testosterone in the body [Ritchason, 1995]. Some studies have shown that women taking the panax variety of ginseng have began showing secondary male traits in as little as 2 months of continued use. It is recommended that women cycle their use of ginseng.

Nitric oxide is a very simple molecule, but it plays an important role in the body. Nitric oxide effects nearly everything from from hair growth to immune function. One of the key effects of Nitric oxide for athletes is that the endothelium (inner lining) of blood vessels uses nitric oxide to signal the surrounding smooth muscle to relax, thus resulting in vasodilation and increasing blood flow.

Typically the body bio-synthesizes nitric oxide endogenously from L-arginine, oxygen, and nicotinamide adenine dinucleotide phosphate. However, some studies have shown that Panax ginseng also promotes endogenous nitric oxide production. One study showed that the ginsenosides Rg1, through endogenous nitric oxide production, induced a protection against left ventricular hypertrophy [Jiang, Deng Et al, 2010]. This typically develops as a response to some factors, such as high blood pressure, that requires the left ventricle to work harder. As a result of the increased work, the walls of the chamber grow thicker, lose elasticity and eventually may fail to pump with as much force as a healthy heart. Humans with atherosclerosis, diabetes, or hypertension often show impaired nitric oxide pathways.

It is no coincidence that the ginsenosides in both *Panax ginseng* and *Panax quinquefolium* are very effective in the treatment of metabolic syndrome. Metabolic Syndrome was first introduced as a concept in 1923 by Dr. Kylin. However, it did not get much coverage until Dr. Reaven introduced his Syndrome X in the late 1980s. There are 6 basic criteria for Metabolic Syndrome diagnosis: hyperglycemia, insulin resistance, central obesity, hypertension, elevated triglycerides, and decreased high-density lipoprotein cholesterol. Ginseng has proven effective for anti-hypoglycemia, insulin sensitization, islet protection, anti-obesity, and anti-oxidative. Energy expenditure is enhanced through the thermogenesis[8] effect of ginseng [Jun Yin, Hanjie Zhang & Jianping Ye, 2008].

Ginseng is one of the key herbs used in the treatment of Type 2 diabetes. Studies in both China and Korea, have shown that an extract of ginseng used regularly reduced fasting blood glucose levels and significantly improved insulin sensitivity. In addition to glucose metabolism, ginseng has also shown effective in regulating lipid metabolism. An overall reduction in cholesterol and triglyceride levels in the liver has been seen in both animal and human studies. Its ability to regulate lipid and glucose metabolism, as well as assist in weight loss through thermogenesis makes the use of this herb beneficial in the treatment of metabolic syndrome related disorders.

One of the most over looked properties of Ginseng is its anticancer properties. However a quick look at the PubMed website reveals no less than 450 articles on the effects of ginseng and ginsenosides on cancer. These studies show that the anti-inflammatory, chemo-preventive, and anti-tumor properties [Cui, Yong Et al, 2006] are the key to ginseng being used to decrease such cancers as pharynx, liver, pancreas, colon, breast, and leukemia. In fact some studies show that the ginsenosides in ginseng cause

---

[8] Def. *thermogenesis* - the production of heat in the body typically through oxidation.

apoptosis of breast cancer cells [Wang, Chong-Zie, Et al, 2008],
colon cancer cells [Wang, Chong-Zie, Et al, 2009], and human
leukemia cells[Cho, Sung-Hee, Et al. 2009].

Chronic inflammation is bad for health in humans. In fact,
numerous studies have linked chronic inflammation as a contributing
factor in cancer. Ginseng has been shown to work as an anti-
inflammatory molecule that targets key players in the inflammation to
cancer sequence such as inflammatory cytokines, nitric oxide
synthases, and toll like receptors [Hofseth and Wargovich, 2007].

Ginseng is one of the most effective adaptogens of the tonic
herbs. It has measurable amounts of germanium, providing energy to
all the body systems. It aids in digestion, promotes regeneration of
the body suffering from stress and fatigue, and has been known to
aid in the rebuilding of body strength. Ginseng supports adrenal
function, reduces stress, and regulates blood sugar. It aids in the
recovery of numerous ailments. Ginseng may be a true panacea.

Wayne A. Pedranti

CHAPTER 9: ASTRAGALUS - *ASTRAGALUS MEMBRANCEUS*

Ginseng may be considered by many to be the father of all tonics. Although it is classified by the Chinese as a chi tonic, it can be used to tonify any genuine deficiency whether it be chi, yang, yin, or blood. However, astragalus is one of the most powerful herbs for the immune system. Although it has most often been used for the purpose of boosting the immune system and aiding digestion, it is also used to counteract the effects of radiation and chemotherapy in cancer patients. In fact, it is used extensively in China for that purpose.

The main constituents of *Astragalus membranceus* include polysaccharides, saponins, flavonoids, amino acids, and trace mineral elements. The polysaccharides fraction F3 has been shown to play an important role in the immunomodulatory action of Astragalus. There are several saponin compounds referred to as astragalosides I – VII. There are eight different flavonoids in Astragalus. Astragalus is a source of gamma-aminobutyric acid (GABA) and L-canavanine. There are several minerals found in the root including zinc, iron, copper, magnesium, manganese, calcium, potassium, sodium, cobalt, and silver. In addition, several organic compounds have been isolated. All these contribute to *Astragalus membranceus* being the immune booster it is.

One way that *Astragalus membranceus* modulates the immune system is through the digestive system. From a Traditional Chinese Medicine point of view, overeating of cold, raw foods, or prolonged fasting can damage the digestive system and bring about a lack of the vital enzymes needed to break down fat. This directly leads to an overweight condition, and the accumulation of fat leads to a stagnation and toxic condition that may be an underlying cause of disease. This results in deficiency of Spleen Yang. As Astragalus is a spleen tonic, it stimulates the digestive system to aid the digestion of fat [Tierra, 1988]. This is evident in modern western study in that Astragalus is known to increase the flow of bile and digestive fluids. According to Michael Tierra N.D., Astragalus taken daily over a period of weeks and months will restore spleen yang, aid assimilation and digestion, and eliminate excess fluid.

Astragalus is rich in polysaccharides that basically are the main nutrient of our bodies. Astragalus supports the immune system at a very deep level. It begins with the increase in stem cells in the bone marrow and lymph tissue [Monograph, 2003]. It encourages and strengthens the function of the T-cells. These white blood cells seek out and destroy foreign invaders in the body . This ability to restore the T-cell activity is one of the leading reasons why *Astragalus membranceus* is used to compliment standard cancer treatments in China [Wu, Ping Et al, 2009]. Astragalus has been shown to increase the resistance to the immunosuppressive effects of chemotherapy drugs and has drastically increased the life expectancy of patients choosing this method of treatment.

In addition to the protective effects of Astragalus to chemotherapy, it also has anti-tumorous properties. A sample of human colon adenocarcinoma cell HT-29 was exposed to a standardized extract of astragalus saponins [Mandy, M.Y. Tin, Et al.

2007]. The research found that astragalus extract induced apoptosis in the HT-29 cells 48 to 72 hours after exposure. They concluded that Astragalus saponins could inhibit human colon cancer cell growth both in vitro and in vivo.

Astragalus has anti-viral properties. It has been shown to reduce and help prevent colds, influenza, bronchitis, mononucleosis, pneumonia, and infections by the coxsackie B virus [Winston and Maimes, 2007]. In a double blind clinical trial, 235 patients with cervicitis associated with the human papillomavirus were given either *Astragalus membranceus* or a placebo. Patients using astragalus showed striking improvements especially when taken in synergy with standard interferon treatment [Monograph, 2003].

Extracorporeal shock wave lithotripsy has become the most accepted treatment for upper urinary tract calculi (ie kidney stones). This treatment of using high energy shock waves is generally perceived as safe, but often results in renal vascular and tubular injury. Originally, it was thought that this type of injury was directly related to the shock waves. Recently, studies have indicated the role of free radicals in renal damage induced by high energy shock waves. Vascular injury causes areas of tissue ischemia (restriction of blood supply). These areas become susceptible to free radical production as reperfusion occurs.

Astragalus is already known to have a definite protective effect against cerebral and renal ischemia reperfusion injury. In a study on rabbits, it was found that *Astragalus membranceus* when given prior to the application of high energy shock waves significantly reduced renal tubule injury mediated by free radicals in the kidney of the rabbit [Shen Et al., 2005].

Other studies have confirmed that Astragalus works as an antioxidant. This protection is contributed for the most part to the flavonoids and saponin found in *Astragalus membranceus*. These can significantly inhibit the membrane lipid peroxidation by the super oxide (O_2), Hydrogen peroxide (H_2O_2), and ultraviolet rays. Astragalus demonstrates inhibitory effects on oxidative stress.

The saponins (particularly Astragaloside IV) contained in *Astragalus membranceus* have a positive effect on the cardiovascular system. Astragalus is an anti-clotting agent. It also has been known to have vasodilating properties that helps prevent coronary heart disease by increasing circulation.

Very little direct research has been made on the effects of *Astragalus membranceus* on athletic performance. However, there are several aspects of Astragalus that may prove beneficial to athletes especially when combined with other adaptogens. First and foremost, Astragalus works as a tonic to the immune system. Strenuous exercise is known to decrease the immune function of the body. Secondly, Astragalus has been demonstrated to increase energy through the reduction of toxicity in the liver. Astragalus combats fatigue by nourishing the adrenals. Astragalus is a heart tonic that lowers blood pressure and reduces fatigue to the heart. It also dilates the blood vessels allowing blood to carry more oxygen to hungry cells. Astragalus has many properties that could benefit an athlete. Because it is a powerful immune-stimulating herb, Astragalus should be used throughout the year.

CHAPTER 10: ADAPTOGENIC HERBS IN COMBINATION AND SYNERGY

It is common practice for herbalists to use multi-herb formulas instead of simple single herb remedies. These single herb remedies are common place as folklore or home remedies. The therapeutic effect of a single herb may not be strong enough, but when added to the effect of a second herb, the therapeutic effect may be exactly what is needed. Nearly all herbal systems including Chinese, Ayurvedic, and Thomsonian rely on the synergistic properties of herbal combinations. Adaptogenic herbs are no different.

Astragalus membranceus is one of the greatest immune stimulating herbs, however, it is rarely used by itself. By combining Astragalus with other herbs, a quite different effect can be achieved. A good example of this is a Chinese treatment for anemia. According to Michael Tierra ND, in Traditional Chinese Medicine, Chi is part of the yang, while the blood is part of the yin. Since the yang and the yin are rooted together, in order to improve one, it is necessary to strengthen the other. That is why for Anemia, Astragalus the chi tonic is combined with Dong quai the actual blood tonic. Further examples show when Astragalus is combined with chuan xiong, an effective treatment for type 2 diabetes is achieved [Winston & Maimes, 2007].

Another adaptogen that often works best when combined with other herbs or adaptogens is Asian ginseng (*Panax ginseng*). Ginseng is often too warming or stimulating, and may lead to insomnia or even heart palpitations. However, when combined with Astragalus or Licorice Root, it becomes less overstimulating and simultaneously increases its sphere of influence.

Early on in his research, Dr. Brekhman MD, the father of modern adaptogenic research, discovered that adaptogenic herbs worked best when combined. Using *Eleutherococcus senticosus* as his chief herb, Dr. Brekhman devised a combination of herbs that he considered most effective. This combination was given in the former USSR to athletes, pilot, cosmonauts, and other workers to relieve the symptoms of stress and improve overall performance. This combination of adaptogens was referred to simply as Prime One. It is accepted as a medicinal agent in Russia and contains: *Eleutherococcus senticosus, Schisandra chinensis, Rhaponticum carthamoides, Rhodiola rosea, Aralia mandshurica, Glycyrrhiza uralensis* (Ural Licorice Root), *Rosa majalis* (Cinnamon Rose), and MA Complex (the still secret ingredient - a combination of adaptogens and molasses). Prime one is thought to be partially responsible for the dominance of the USSR Olympic Team in the 1970's and 80's

In another study in Sweden, it was found that a simple combination of *Eleutherococcus senticosus, Schisandra chinensis,* and *Rhodiola rosea* was very effective. During a study of literature, the researchers found that these three adaptogens had pharmacological profiles that were unique but similar in their stress protective action [Panossian & Wikman, 2010]. They also found in the same publication that nematodes (*C. elegans*) when given this combination had a 129% increase in life span. In another test on humans, it was found that when given this combination, there was a significant increase in performance and mental working capacity within 30 minutes of taking it, and the effects lasted for 4 to 6 hours [Panossian and Wagner, 2005]. Adaptogens can, and are, taken as a single herb with good results. However, just like all herbs, they can be combined with other adaptogens or non-adaptogenic herbs. This is done to increase or improve their function. David Winston, author of the Book Adaptogens: Herbs for Strength, Stamina, and Stress Relief, suggests that the adaptogenic herbs mentioned in this paper can be combined as follows:

1. *Eleutherococcus senticosus* combines well with nervines and antidepressants such as fresh milky oat, mimosa bark, hawthorn, and St. John's wort;

2. Red (*Panax ginseng*) Asian ginseng can be combined with licorice and reishi to treat Addison's Disease (adrenal depletion);

3. *Rhodiola rosea* combines well with amla, cordyceps, and reishi to prevent and treat altitude sickness and jet lag;

4. Asian ginseng combines with licorice and schisandra to relieve shortness of breath and asthma;

5. Schisandra combined with prince seng and dang shen helps to reduce wheezing and asthma. When taken over long periods of time, it can reduce the fatigue associated with chronic fatigue syndrome;

6. For speeding up the recovery from head trauma injury, rhodiola combined with holy basil and another nootropic such as ginkgo can be used;

7. Astragalus combined with hawthorn and rhodiola can enhance cardiac function and reduce angina pain;

8. Asian ginseng, rhodiola, ashwagandha and cordyceps when combined shows significant benefits for men suffering from erectile dysfunction. This formula has also been known to enhance male fertility.

Wayne A. Pedranti

CHAPTER 11: CONCLUSION

Adaptogens have been used for thousands of years in China and India. Their use has demonstrated a beneficial stress protective action that is related to the regulation of homeostasis. This is done by supporting the HPA axis and regulating the key mediators of the stress response. Adaptogenic herbs support the body in a non-specific way that is counter to the one drug one problem paradigm.

It is evident that adaptogens have specific therapeutic effects related to stress induced or stress related disorders. They can also work to improve the quality of life when used in combination with other standard treatments such as chemotherapy. Adaptogens are extremely beneficial for the elderly suffering from age related disorders. Adaptogens are beneficial for improving athletic performance by reducing fatigue and aiding in recovery. These effects have been most pronounced on untrained or beginning athletes.

Wayne A. Pedranti

WORKS CITED

1. Abidoff, Dr. Musa, and Ramazanov, Dr. Zakir, "*Rhodiola rosea*: The Herbal Heavyweight from Russia" Muscle Development, January (2003)
2. Abidov M, Et al "Effects of Extracts from Rhodiola rosea and Rhodiola crenulata Roots on ATP Content in Mitochondria of Skeletal Muscles" Bulletin of Experimental Biological Medicine, December (2003) 585-7
3. Boon-Niermeijer, E.K. Et al, "Phyto-Adaptogen Protect Against Environmental Stress-induced Death of Embryos from Freshwater Snail Lymnea stagnalis." Phytomedicine, Vol 7(5) (2000) 389-399
4. Bompa,Tudor O. & Haff, G. Gregory, Periodization: Theory and Methodology of Training, Champaign Illinois: Human Kinetics, 2009.
5. Cao, Shehua Et al, "Evaluation of Anti-athletic Fatigue Activity of *Schizandra chinesis* Aqueous Extract in Mice." African Journal of Pharmacy and Pharmacology, Vol. 3(11) (2009)
6. Cho, Sung-Hee Et al, "Compound K, A Metabolite of Ginseng Saponin, Induces Apoptosis Via Caspase-8-Dependent Pathway in HL-60 Human Leukemia Cells." BMC Cancer, Vol. 9 (2009)

7. Chu-Bing, Tan Et al, "Protective Effects of Salidroside on Endothelial Cell Apoptosis Induced by Cobalt Chloride." Biological Pharmaceutical Bulletin, (2009) 1359 – 1363

8. Colgan, Michael. Optimum Sports Nutrition: Your Competitive Edge. New York: Advanced Research Press, 1993.

9. Cui, yong, Et al, " Association of Ginseng Use with Survival and Quality of Life Among Breast Cancer Patients." American Journal of Epidemiology February (2006)

10. De Bock, K Et al "Acute *Rhodiola rosea* Intake Can Improve Endurance Exercise Performance." International journal of Sports Nutrition and Exercise Metabolism June (2004).

11. Deng, Jiang Et al "Role of Nitric Oxide in Ginsenoside Rg1 Induced Protection Against Left Ventricular Hypertrophy Produced by Abdominal Aorta Coarctation in Rats." Biological Pharmaceutical Bulletin Vol 33(4), 2010.

12. Hofseth, Lorne and Wargovich, Michael, "Inflamation, Cancer, and Targets of Ginseng." The Journal of Nutrition, (2007)

13. Holly, Cory. Certified Sports Adviser Education Program Module 4: Dietary Supplement Review. Vancouver Canada, Cory Holly Institute, 2007.

14. Jun Yin, Hanjie Zhang, and Jianping ye, "Traditional Chinese Medicine in Treatment of Metabolic Syndrome." Endocrine Metabolic Immune Disorder Drug Targets, June 2008.

15. Kelly, Gregory S, ND, "Rhodiola rosea: A Possible Plant Adaptogen." Alternative Medicine Review, Volume 6, Number 3, 2001.

16. Khanum, Farhath Et al, "Rhodiola rosea, A Versitile Adaptogen." Comprehensive Reviews in Food Science and Food Safety, Vol 4, (2005) 55-62

17. Kuo, Jip Et al, "The effects of Eight Weeks of Supplementation with *Eleutherococcus senticosus* on Endurance Capacity and Metabolism in Human." Chinese Journal of Physiology, (2010)

18. Lee Jia, Yuqing Zhao, and Xing-Jie Liang, "Current Evaluation of the Mellenium Phytomedicine – Ginseng (II): Collected Chemical Entities, Modern Pharmacology, and Clinical Applications from Trdaitional Chinese Medicine." Current Medical Chemistry, 16(22), (2009) 2924 – 2942 .

19. Mandy, M.Y. Tin, Et al. "Astragalus Saponins Induce Growth Inhibitions and Apoptosis in Human Colon Cancer Cells and Tumor Xenograft." Carcinogenesis Vol 28 no. 6 1347-1355, (2007)
20. "Monograph: Astragalus *membranceus*." Alternative Medicine Review, Vol. 8 Number 1, (2003)
21. "Monograph: *Eleutherococcus senticosus*." Alternative Medicine Review, Vol. 11 Number 2, (2006)
22. "Monograph: *Panax ginseng*." Alternative Medicine Review, Vol. 14 Number 2, (2009)
23. Pan, Si-Yuan Et al. "Ethanol Extract of Fructus Schisandrae Decreases Hepatic Triglyceride Level in Mice Fed with a High Fat/Cholesterol Diet, with Attention to Acute Toxicity." eCAM (2009)
24. Panossian, A. Et al. "Effects of Heavy Physical Exercise and Adaptogens on Nitric Oxide Content in Human Saliva.." Phytomedicine Vol 6(1) (1999)
25. Panossian, A. and Wagner, H. "Stimulating Effect of Adaptogens: An Overview with Particular Reference to Their Efficacy Following Single Dose Administration." Phytotherapy Research (2005)
26. Panossian, Alexander and Wikman, Georg "Effect of Adaptogens on the Central Nervous System." Arquivos Brasileiros de Fitomedicina Clientifica Vol.3 Num. 1 (2005).
27. Panossian, Alexander and Wikman, Georg "Effects of Adaptogens on the Central Nervous System and the Molecular Mechanisms Associated with Their Stress Protective Activity." Pharmaceuticals (2010) 188-224.
28. Panossian, A., Wikman, G. and Wagner, H "Plant Adaptogens III. Earlier and More Recent Aspects and Concepts on Their Mode of Action." Phytomedicine Vol.6 Num. 4 (1999).
29. Parisi, A. Et al "Effects of Chronic *Rhodiola rosea* Supplementation on Sport Performance and Antioxidant Capacity in Trained Male: preliminary results." Journal of Sports Medicine and Physical Fitness March (2010).
30. Ritchason N.D., Jack. The Little Herb Encyclopedia: The Hand book of Natures Remedies for a Healthier Life. Pleasant Grove Utah: Woodland Health Books, 1995.

31. Seely, Dugald and Singh, Rana "Adaptogenic Potential of a Polyherbal Natural Health Product: Report on a Longitudinal Clinical Trial." eCAM 4(3) (2007) 375-380.
32. Selye, Hans "The Nature of Stress." Basal Facts (1985)
33. Shen, G birr Wu, Et al. "Astragalus membranceus Reduces Free Radical-Mediated Injury to Renal Tubules in Rabbits Receiving High Energy Shock Waves." Chinese Medical Journal (2005)
34. Tierra, Michael. Planetary Herbology. Twin Lakes Wisconsin: Lotus Press, 1988.
35. Udinstev, SN and Schakhov, VP, "Decrease of Cyclophosphamide heamatoxicity by *Rhodiola rosea* Root Extract in Mice with Ehrlich and Lewis Transplantable Tumors." European Journal of Cancer 27(9) (1991) 1182.
36. Voces, J., Et al, "Ginseng Administration Protects Skeletal Muscle from Oxidative Stress Induced by Acute Exercise in Rats." Brazilian Journal of Medical Biological Research Vol 31(12) (2004).
37. WADA "The 2010 Prohibited List, International Standard." World Anti Doping Agency, 2010.
38. Wang, Chong-Zhi, Et al, "The Mitochondrial Pathway id Involved in American Ginseng Induced Apoptosis of SW-480 Colon Cancer Cells." Oncology Rep Vol 28(5A) (2008) 2545-2551.
39. Wang, Chong-Zhi, Et al, "Chemopreventive Effects of Heat-Processed *Panax quinquefolius* Root on Human Breast Cancer Cells." Anticancer Research Vol 21(3) (2009) 577-584
40. Wang, Rubin. Et al "A Survey of Chinese Herbal Ingredients With Liver Protection Activities." Chinese Medicine May (2007).
41. Winston, David and Maimes, Steven. Adaptogens herbs for strength, stamina, and stress relief. Rochester Vermont: Healing Arts Press, 2007.
42. wu, Ping Et al. "Traditional Chinese Medicine in the Treatment of Hepatocellular Cancers: a Systematic Review and Meta-Analysis." Journal of Experimental and Clinical Cancer Research, (2009).
43. Xie, Jing-Teng Et al. "In Vitro and In Vivo Anticancer Effects of American Ginseng Berry: Exploring

Representative Compounds." Biological Pharmaceutical
Bulletin, Vol 32(9) (2009) 1552-1558.

Wayne A. Pedranti

INDEX

creatine phosphate, 20, 24

A

adenocarcinoma, *52*
adrenal glands, 5, 6, 34
adrenocorticotropic hormone, 6
amenorrhea, *32, 34*
Andenosine Triphosphate, 20, 24
antioxidant, *30, 38, 46, 53*
anxiety, 3, 7, 15, 37, 38
autoimmune disease, 3

B

balance
    nitrogen, *25*
Brekhman. Isreal I., 12, 20, 56

C

cardiovascular disease, 3
cholesterol, *39, 48*
corticotropin-releasing hormone, 6
cortisol, 6, 7, 8, 9, 15, 24, 25, 40

D

depression, 3, 34, 38
diabetes, 3, 8, 28, 39, 47, 48, 56

E

endocrine, *11, 17, 27, 32, 34, 37*

F

fatigue, 9, 15, 16, 20, 26, 27, 28, 29, 34, 40, 41, 45, 46, 49, 54, 57, 59
fibromyalgia, 3, 28

G

gastrointestinal ulcerations, 3
General Adaptation Syndrome, 7, 19, 40
ginsenoside, *13, 43, 44, 45, 47, 48*

glutathione, *38*

H

hippocampus, 6
hyperglycemia, *48*
hypothalamus, 5, 6

I

inflammation, *7*, *46*, *49*
inflammatory bowel disease, 3

L

Lazarev, Nikolai, 12
L-canavanine, *51*

N

nitrogen, *24*, *25*

O

Olympics, *20*, *33*

P

pituitary gland, 5, 6
Prime One, *20*, *56*

S

schizophrenia, 3, 28, 35
Selye. Hans, 5, 7, 64
stimulants, 15, 16, 32, 34
sympathetic nervous system, 6, 15, 34
Syndrome X, *48*

T

thermogenesis, *48*
Tierra. Michael, *39*, *52*, *55*, *64*
tonic, *11*, *15*, *16*, *26*, *43*, *49*, *51*, *52*, *54*, *55*

ABOUT THE AUTHOR

Wayne Pedranti is an Aerospace Engineer and cyclist who began his interest in natural health after heavy metal toxicity began effecting his competitive performance. He is a Naturopath, Master Herbalist, Cycling Coach, and Track and Field Coach. He currently runs Naturally Sports and Wellness with his wife Johanna.